FIRST AID KITS FOR HOME AND AUTO

Essential Gear to Survive until Help Arrives

R. BRYAN SIMON, RN, FAWM

Ourea Publishing

Ourea Publishing

PO Box 405, Fayetteville, WV 25840-6193

www.oureapublishing.com

FIRST AID KITS FOR HOME AND AUTO

ISBN: 978-1-7336232-1-6

Notices:

Knowledge and best practices in medicine are constantly changing as new research and experience enhance our understanding of methods, treatment, and professional practice. Practitioners and untrained persons must always rely on their own experience and knowledge in using any information, methods, or materials described within this text. All persons must consider the safety to themselves and others when using any technique, tool, or medication described within and are advised to check current information on proper use, dosage, administration, and contraindications for all drugs mentioned herein. Certain techniques and items described in this text require training and should not be used or attempted without proper first aid or medical training. Attempt no procedures outside of your skill level. The author and publisher have made every effort to ensure that the information included within this text is as accurate and up-to-date as possible. To the fullest extent of the law, neither the publisher nor the author assume any liability for any personal injury and/or damage to persons or property, or death as a matter of products liability, negligence, or otherwise, or from any use or operations of any methods, products, instructions, or ideas contained in this text.

Cover Illustration: Mark Quire, quiregraphics.com

FIRST AID KITS FOR HOME AND AUTO

This book is dedicated to my mother, a true heroine, who taught me by example that preparation and the determination to succeed can overcome any obstacle.

Foreword

My own personal story as a medical professional began with a simple realization. The more adventures I wanted to have, and the more I matured in my wish to take care of those I loved, the more medical training I realized I needed to have. For me, this led to a career in medicine, and an interest in extending my care to professional relationships and teaching others about first aid and EMS medical care. But for most, this realization points to a simpler yet still exceptionally effective goal: building and maintaining a first aid medical kit.

It has long been considered a fundamental tenet of emergency preparation that one should have a first aid kit. We are a species that lives within a threatening environment regardless of our location, and means to manage risk and actual injury or illness is always important. Our risk profile has grown even more changed in the 21st century, with threats of increased weather events as our climate changes and ever more credible threats of terrorism and violence in the United States and internationally. These changes are coupled with a dizzying new array of first aid products and treatment principles; a growing realization that in disasters both major and minor we are likely to be "on our own" for a period of time without expectation of governmental help; and a growing understanding in the EMS and emergency management community that first aid is in fact the most important intervention for many immediate life threats. All this can make the task of preparing for medical emergencies seem both more important and more daunting than ever before.

Bryan Simon is the man to lead you out of that state of paralysis and inaction.

Mr. Simon has a remarkable professional story. He joined the service, graduated from Ranger School and was for a time the youngest infantry company commander in the US Army before moving his professional path on to nursing. He is not only a clinically active Operating Room nurse, but is also the first nurse in the world (along with his wife) to earn a Master's Degree in Mountain Medicine as well as a Diploma in Mountain Medicine. As the co-founder of Vertical Medicine Resources, he has run medical training programs around the world for years. I've been witness myself to countless sessions he has run specifically training students on building medical kits. For these many achievements he has been named a Master Fellow of the Adventurers and Explorers Guild (also the first nurse to earn this credential) and a Fellow of the

Academy of Wilderness Medicine. Beyond his academic and clinical skills, he is also an accomplished climber and international traveler who has logged miles on the ground in nearly every part of the world and an accomplished medical writer of both books and columns.

The pages you are about to read contain pure distilled wisdom: the logistical savvy of an infantry officer, the operational experience of an international traveler and mountaineer, the academic know-how of a credentialed subject matter master, the communication abilities of an accomplished writer, and the clinical experience of a seasoned nurse.

In this book, Mr. Simon makes an interesting and quite true point: it is difficult, if not impossible, to find a medical kit that is truly customized to your own needs. Every person reading this book has a uniquely different set of environmental, personal, and recreational or professional needs that drive slightly different priorities for medical planning. Mr. Simon works from the assumption that any kit, whether built from scratch or starting from a commercial project, will need to be adapted to your own individual needs. He will be meticulously and expertly leading you through various considerations for building and continuing to adapt your own medical kit.

Some of you may find that this journey piques an interest in further training. In this regard, the sky is the limit, and I encourage you to seek quality course work that further reinforces and expands your interest. You may find your kit grows in conjunction with this training, or becomes more refined with your growing expertise. And yet the most important growth, as Mr. Simon himself points out in this book, is your own knowledge, experience, and clinical intelligence. As your confidence grows, you will find that while at one time your priority was what you should carry and then learning how to use it, you will cross a threshold where your priority becomes what you know, and then learning what you need to carry to support that knowledge.

Your medical kit is an intrinsic part of that equation, regardless of which side of that growth threshold you find yourself on. With the help of this book, you are well-positioned to begin engaging in this world, or moving your current engagement much further forward. It will be fun, and can also be one of the most significant projects you take on… as it is no exaggeration whatsoever to think that your health and life itself, and that of your loved ones, may depend on the preparation you do here. Carry on, and with the help of this book, may all your misadventures be manageable and result in great stories at the end of the journey!

Seth Collings Hawkins, MD, FACEP, FAEMS, MFAWM, MFAEG

Morganton, North Carolina

1

Introduction

Introduction

I hope you never need the knowledge contained within this book. I had hoped to never use a first aid kit in an emergency. Unfortunately, that has not been the case. As a US Army infantry officer and now as a registered nurse who specializes in wilderness medicine, I have had to use my first aid and medical training often…too often. Having the essential gear necessary to react and care for someone after an accident is crucial and may be the most important thing you ever do. This book is the first step of preparation and I applaud you for taking it.

The modern world has insulated us from many of the dangers of the past. The United States health care system, while expensive, is one of the best in the world, and science has continued to find cures for diseases and solutions to once commonplace dangers. There is a continual technological march towards safer automobiles, homes, and workplaces but there remain hazards to ourselves and our family's health and well-being.

According to accident data from the Insurance Institute for Highway Safety (IIHS) (www.iihs.org), an average of 102 Americans died each day due to automobile accidents in 2017 (37,133 total deaths).[1] This is down from the over 40,000 deaths recorded yearly between 2000-2007. The statistics are more dramatic when considering deadly automobile accidents throughout the world. The World Health Organization (WHO) estimates that 1.24 million people die each year in road traffic accidents. That equates to almost 3,400 deaths each day.[2] Injury data for automobile accidents are even more dire with the United States Centers for Disease Control (CDC) estimating that 2.3 million people are taken to emergency departments (ED) on a yearly basis for an average of 6,301 injuries from motor vehicle crashes each day.[3] **Today, as you are reading this book, Americans will suffer roughly 6,300 injuries and 100 deaths due to automobile accidents.**

Information regarding accidental injury and death in the home are somewhat more difficult to estimate, but the CDC determined that there were 30.8 million unintended injuries that resulted in visits to emergency departments and 161,374 unintentional deaths in 2015.[4] These could have occurred anywhere, not just in the home or workplace. If you remove the averages related to motor vehicle injury and death discussed above, that amount is reduced to 28.5 million unintentional injuries and approximately 120,000 unintentional injury related deaths. **This averages to over 78,000 ED visits and 442 deaths due to unintentional injury each day.**

So how do we avoid being a part of these statistics? Well, living in a safety bubble is certainly a solution, but not one that is practical. We cannot insulate ourselves from every danger but we can prepare, mitigate risks, and have the knowledge and materials needed to address injuries due to a motor vehicle accident, or due to a fall, slip of a knife, or any of a number of accidents that can occur at home.

Beyond being careful and aware of dangers in our environment, the key is to be prepared, with knowledge and materials, to address unintentional injuries whenever they do occur. Within these pages, you will find the detailed information that you will need to gather the items and build a first aid kit that is useful to you and your family. And while having the needed first aid items is a useful first step, having knowledge in first aid techniques is also essential. Chapter 8 discusses in detail the many classes and programs available to give you the necessary skills and confidence to treat injuries until help arrives.

Why build a kit?

This text discusses the relevant first aid supplies needed to address the most common injuries in the home and in the event of a motor vehicle accident. The primary purpose of this book is to explain the need for a kit that is purpose-driven, while taking into account personal and environmental variables. It is important to remember that there is no universally suitable first aid kit for sale today. **The only perfect kit for you is the one that has what you need at the time you need it.**

There are hundreds of pre-packaged first aid kits on the market today, but most are woefully short of the essential items needed in a crisis. Instead, they are packed with items that are poorly manufactured and often downright useless in a true emergency. While these kits might be perfect for a minor cut or scrape, an unexpected headache, or a mildly sprained ankle, most don't contain the materials needed to address the needs of a larger bleeding laceration or other more severe injuries. The purchase of a prepackaged kit might "check the box" on your to-do list but might not have the needed items when an accident happens. A comprehensive and customized kit, developed after a careful consideration of common injuries/illnesses and environmental risk, and combined with the knowledge to employ the stocked items, can be the critical factor in caring for an injured person.

In addition to the issue of availability of key material, commercially available kits are also often comprised of poorly made materials. Having taught scores of first aid and wilderness medicine classes, it continually amazes me to find bandages with no adhesive, ice packs that will not get cold, and alcohol pads that are dry. As the old adage goes, "You get what you pay for." You, your loved ones, and others who you may have to care for in an emergency deserve the best care you can provide. That begins with a comprehensive kit that can address immediate needs of the injured and keep them alive until they reach definitive care.

Will it be expensive?

Will it be expensive? Surprisingly not. In the current commercial reality of the United States, it is possible to buy the materials needed to put together a comprehensive kit at a relatively low cost. Between online retailers, local big box stores, and discount shops in your area, all of the needed materials will be available for a reasonable price. Likely, once you have read this text, you will see the need to have a number of kits available for you and your family's use in your home, in all of your automobiles, at a vacation home, and at your workplace. You might consider working with other family members or neighbors, church groups, or other social clubs about purchasing items in bulk and splitting costs to reduce expenses even more. Other ideas include building and giving first aid kits to family members for birthdays or Christmas gifts. Nothing says "I care about you" more than that!

While controlling cost is a factor, it is important to recognize the need for quality. After all, one of the principle reasons for building a kit on your own is to have quality materials that do what you intend them to when you need them. So, spending a little more for a better product should remain a high priority. Even so, this can be done on a budget!

So why the guide?

This guide provides a quality reference by distilling the latest and best medical advice available related to common injuries to determine what items are needed to treat these injuries in a first aid scenario. This is done using the latest evidence-based medicine and authoritative consensus guidelines pertaining to first aid kits. When practical, this guide includes these primary materials as references at the end of each chapter for you to review if interested. Additionally, you will see numerous references throughout the text indicating material and instruments that require training to use properly. Gear without associated knowledge is often unusable and, in some cases, dangerous. Classes in basic first aid and cardiopulmonary resuscitation (CPR) are common and are usually very reasonably priced. **A customized, well-stocked first aid kit and the knowledge to use it correctly could mean the difference between life and death.**

Let's get building!

References

1. Insurance Institute for Highway Safety. 2018. General Statistics – yearly snapshot. Available at www.iihs.org/iihs/topics/t/general-statistics/fatalityfacts/overview-of-fatality-facts. Accessed January 13, 2019.

2. World Health Organization. 2013. Global Road

Safety Infographic. Available at www.who.int/violence_injury_prevention/road_safety_status/2013/facts/en/. Accessed January 12, 2019.

3. U.S. Centers for Disease Control (CDC). 2016. Motor Vehicle Injuries. Available at www.cdc.gov/winnablebattles/report/motor.html. Accessed January 12, 2019.

4. U.S. Centers for Disease Control (CDC). 2016. Accidents or Unintentional Injuries. Available at www.cdc.gov/nchs/fastats/accidental-injury.htm. Accessed January 16, 2019.

2

Risk Assessment and Considerations

Risk Assessment and Considerations

The idea of conducting a risk assessment is common in nearly all industries from healthcare to construction but is not often thought of within the context of home safety. Risk assessment, put simply, is a systematic process of evaluating the potential risks that may be involved in a projected activity or undertaking. Therefore, the first step in creating a customized and comprehensive first aid kit is to move through a logical sequence of steps that identify common injuries and illnesses, common hazards within the environment, and an assessment of the knowledge needed to act if these injuries or illnesses occur. The table below lists the steps to consider within this process and the remainder of the chapter will focus on moving through each stage.

Risk Assessment Steps

1. Identify common injuries and illnesses
2. Decide who might be harmed and how
3. Evaluate risk of injury
4. Decide on FA kit contents and knowledge deficiency
5. Stock FA kit and gain needed knowledge

Step 1: Identification of most common types of injuries or illnesses

According to the CDC, the two most common causes of unintentional non-fatal injuries for all age groups are classified as either "unintentional falls" or unintentional "struck by/against."[1] The latter category would be either hitting or being hit by an object. This grouping does not include motor vehicle accidents, as these are listed as a separate category. Luckily, a well-designed first aid kit will have items that can assist in the care of people injured in these types of accidents.

A broader view of injury causes within the United States is possible by utilizing the CDC's Web-based Injury Statistics Query and Reporting System (WISQARS). This system allows the user to search the most recent injury and death statistical data to identify the most common causes of injury and death. From this information, the top ten leading causes of nonfatal injuries for all persons (age 1-80) are listed below based on the latest available CDC data from 2017.

Top Ten Non-Fatal Injuries – 2017[2]

1. Unintentional Falls
2. Unintentional Struck by/Against
3. Unintentional Overexertion
4. Unintentional Motor Vehicle Accident
5. Unintentional Other (unspecified)
6. Unintentional Cut/Pierce
7. Unintentional Poisoning
8. Other Assault/Struck by/Against
9. Unintentional Other Bite/Sting
10. Unintentional Unknown/Other

The top ten leading causes of death for all persons (age 1-80) are listed below based again on the latest available CDC data from 2017. As you can see many of these are long-term disease processes rather than unintentional injury. While there are items that can be included in first aid kits to assist with some disease processes (e.g. heart disease), the focus of this discussion will be on the third item of the list below: Unintentional Injury.

Top Ten Fatal Injuries/Illnesses – 2017[3]

1. Malignant Neoplasms (Cancer)
2. Heart Disease
3. Unintentional Injury
4. Chronic Respiratory Disease
5. Cerebrovascular event/disease
6. Diabetes Mellitus
7. Suicide
8. Liver disease
9. Nephritis (Kidney inflammation)

10. Septicemia (Infection of the blood stream)

Unintentional injury, while ranking third for fatal injuries and illnesses for the 1-80 age range, actually ranks first for all groups aged 1-44. The list below contains the top ten unintentional injuries for this age range.

Top Ten Unintentional Injuries resulting in Death – 2017[4]

1. Poisoning
2. Motor Vehicle Accident
3. Drowning
4. Fall
5. Fire/Burn
6. Suffocation
7. Other land transport
8. Other/Specified
9. Pedestrian/Other
10. Unspecified

The next five causes include:

11. Natural/environment
12. Other transport
13. Firearm
14. Struck by or against
15. Machinery[4]

Step 2. Decide who might be harmed and how

It is certainly feasible to simply use the information

collected above in step 1 of the risk assessment process, but using the CDC website and database to identify the specific risks for family members by age will allow the user to better identify the dangers for their individual circumstances. The link to access this website is: www.cdc.gov/injury/wisqars/index.html. After clicking on this link and choosing "Non-fatal injury data" or "fatal injury data," you can use the advanced search options to create searches based on sex, age, and ethnicity.

Other important considerations, outside of determining the most common injuries for members of your family, include current medical conditions and specialized activities. Do members of your family have heart disease or any other long-term illnesses? Do your children spend a large amount of time outside or are they involved in contact sports? Does anyone in your family operate motorcycles or off-road vehicles? Do you spend time boating? Are there any other specialized activities that introduce risks not common to the general public?

Step 3. Evaluate risk of injury

The next aspect of this process is to evaluate the risk of injury from the identified common injuries for members of your family based on CDC data in general and your family's specific situation. If you live in a city and rarely drive, your potential involvement in a motor vehicle accident is much lower than for someone who might commute for an hour each day. The same is true with any number of the top ten injuries identified earlier.

The environment in which you will be using these kits is important to consider when evaluating risk. Do you live and work in a desert environment? A cold environment? What are some of the weather hazards in your current area? Do you live near a coast that is subject to hurricane activity, or the Midwest where tornados are a threat? These are the types of questions that must be considered. Examples of items for consideration based on location and unique environmental hazards are included below.

High Temperature Environments

In high temperature environments, you must consider worst case scenarios in order to prepare for any eventuality. Stocking extra water, food, and oral rehydration solutions are some obvious needs in this environment. Having means to purify additional water is a must as is having some type of shelter (if needed) to provide shade. High temperature environments almost always are associated with bright sunlight and thus sunscreen and sunglasses should be included. These items are especially important for a vehicle based first aid kit as a mechanical breakdown in a remote area could result in a long wait for assistance. Additionally, in desert areas, the temperature shift can be extreme and night temperatures can be intensely cold in relation to daytime highs. Additional layers may be needed to stay warm in the event of an unexpected overnight stay.

Cold Temperature Environments

As with high temperatures, the extreme cold can put a

stranded traveler at risk. In addition to extra water and food, extra clothing, additional warm layers and blankets should be included with first aid items whenever traveling. Heat packets and "space blankets" are also good to include as are a few candles and some fire source. In an enclosed vehicle cab a simple candle can raise the temperature a number of degrees.

Remote or Difficult Terrain

Preparation for becoming stranded is essential in extreme remote environments. Extra food, water, clothing, and a means to stay warm/cool should be a part of any first aid kit. Items to be kept in motor vehicles and specialized items depending on environmental considerations are discussed in detail in Chapter 6.

Step 4. Decide on FA kit contents and knowledge deficiency

After identifying the most common injuries based on statistical data, any specialized risks to members of your family, and evaluating these risks based on the environment and any special factors specific to you, the next step is to identify items to include in your first aid kit and where these kits should be located. It is equally important to identify any gaps in knowledge that you or members of your family might have using items in the first aid kit. Chapters 3-7 discuss the details of constructing a kit specific to your needs. Chapter 8 reviews useful classes that provide the education needed to quickly respond to accidents and care for injured persons.

Step 5. Stock first aid kit and acquire the most important tool

The final step in the risk assessment process and the topic of the remainder of this book is the selection of items for first aid kits and associated acquisition of knowledge, based on the information learned from the previous steps of this chapter. You can have the most comprehensive first aid kit in the world, but without the knowledge to utilize its contents, it (and you) will be worthless in an emergency. The most important tool to have in an emergency is KNOWLEDGE!

References

1. U.S. Centers for Disease Control (CDC). 2018. 10 Leading Causes of Nonfatal Injury, United States 2017. Available at webappa.cdc.gov/sasweb/ncipc/nfilead-.html. Accessed January 20, 2019.

2. U.S. Centers for Disease Control (CDC). National Center for Health Statistics (NCHS). 2018. 10 Leading Causes of Nonfatal Injury, United States 2017 (Ages 1-80). Available at webappa.cdc.-gov/sasweb/ncipc/nfilead.html. Accessed January 20, 2019.

3. U.S. Centers for Disease Control (CDC). National Center for Health Statistics (NCHS). 2018. 10 Leading Causes of Death, United States 2017 (Ages 1-80). Avail-

able at webappa.cdc.gov/sasweb/ncipc/nfilead.html. Accessed January 20, 2019.

4. U.S. Centers for Disease Control (CDC). National Center for Health Statistics (NCHS). 2018. United States Unintentional Injuries, Ages 1-44, All Races, Both Sexes Total Deaths. Accessed January 20, 2019.

3

Location, Design, and Organization

Location, Design, and Organization

Now that you have identified the most common types of injuries and illnesses that you and your family may encounter based upon your circumstances and environment, the next step is to decide on the location, design, and organization of first aid kits to meet these needs. This chapter will discuss how to identify locations for first aid kits, the type of container to use for each type of kit, and how best to organize them.

Location

There are a number of factors to consider when deciding on the location for a first aid kit in the home and vehicle. The first element is accessibility. For the home, a kit should be located in an area that allows easy access by all mature members of a family while preventing children from accidentally accessing medications or other items that could cause harm. Many families create two kits in this situation, one that is accessible by adults and another, stocked mainly with adhesive bandages, that children can access.

Many new cars today have an option for inclusion of a first aid kit when purchased from a dealer. In fact, some countries require carrying such a kit and fine drivers if these do not meet a minimum standard. Auto-based first aid kits usually reside in the trunk of the car, and that is one of the worst places for them! As with a home kit, you want to protect the contents by keeping it in a place that is accessible and that equates to the passenger area of a car, sports utility vehicle (SUV), or truck.

A second location factor to consider is protection. First aid kits should be stored in a cool, dark, and dry place. Excessive heat or cold and direct sunlight has the ability to degrade individual components, especially medications. Direct sunlight can begin breakdown of materials both in the kit and even portions of the kit itself, especially if it includes clear plastic dividers. Though convenient, storing a kit under the kitchen or bathroom sink is a bad place due to moisture exposure. In a vehicle, storing kits under the front seats (room permitting) or in a storage compartment work well, though temperature extremes can be difficult to avoid. Some medications degrade at hot temperatures or can freeze. Always follow the directions for each medication to ensure the efficacy of the drug and store these items separately if needed.

To summarize, kits must be quickly accessible in case of emergency, but out of reach of children, and should be protected from extreme variance of temperatures, moisture, and direct sunlight.

Design

There are thousands of containers that can be used to store first aid kits and the only limit in choosing one for your needs is your own creativity. The kit container must have a number of attributes. A container should be able to easily fit all of the contents in an organized manner, it should be able to provide an element of protection to these contents while in storage or in use, its configuration should match its intended use, and it should be easily identifiable.

There is no government guidance related to first aid kits for the home or auto, though the Department of Labor's Occupational Safety and Health Administration (OSHA) uses the American National Standards Institute/International Safety Equipment Association (ANSI/ISEA) guidelines for inclusion of kits and kit contents in the workplace. The specific regulation (ANSI/ISEA Z308 1-2015) last updated in 2015 divides kit types into four categories:

Type I – for use in stationary, indoor settings where the potential for damage of kit supplies due to environmental factors and rough handling is minimal.

Type II – for portable use in indoor settings where the potential for damage of kit supplies due to environmental factors and rough handling is minimal.

Type III – for portable use in mobile, indoor and/or outdoor settings where the potential for damage of kit supplies due to environmental factors is not probable.

Type IV – for portable use in the mobile industries and/or outdoor settings where the potential for damage to kit supplies due to environmental factors and rough handling is significant.[1]

It is possible to purchase these containers online, and the information above will help if you choose to use a certified container as often they are labeled by type without further information (e.g. Type I container).

One of the biggest failings in both commercial and personalized first aid kit containers is that they are too small. Commercialized kits will be very organized when purchased but after adding other necessary supplies or after an initial use they are nearly impossible to put back into order.

A suitable container should be at least 25% larger than the total contents of the kit when fully organized. Once the kit is used for the first time, items will likely not be placed back in an orderly fashion, as obviously, the kit was pulled out for a reason (an emergency!). What is not used will be hurriedly stuffed back in while focusing on the injured person. By having this additional space, even an unorganized kit can have the latches, snaps, or zipper engaged, protecting the remaining items for later use.

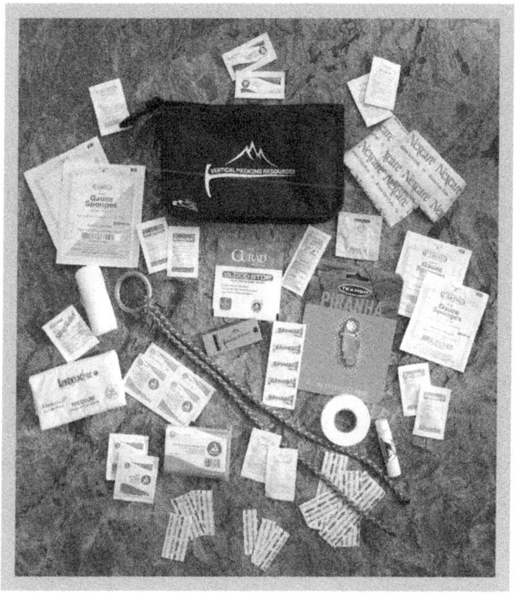

A slightly larger container makes organization much easier.

Protection from the environment in essential to prevent degradation of first aid supplies. Keeping in mind that you will need to protect the contents of the kit from moisture, most people incorporate some type of waterproofing, and often multiple layers of waterproofing in a kit. Additionally, consider using a light-colored material if the container will be exposed to direct sunlight for any amount of time as it will keep the supplies cooler than a darker case.

Choosing a hard-shell case versus a soft case might be wise when focused on protection of supplies. A hard-sided case might not be suitable if portability is a concern. If a kit is likely to stay in one place and rarely be moved, a hard-sided waterproof case, such as the Pelican™ brand cases, or something similar (e.g. a plastic "ammo" can), will protect the kit's contents from nearly any eventuality.

Most commercial kits are easily recognizable as they are typically red and white in color. While the availability of generic red containers is limited, hard cases can be painted, covered in reflective tape, or otherwise distinguished in a manner as to make them easily recognizable. The same can be done with soft cases, using thread, ribbon, or patches.

Organization

Kits should be organized in a manner that allows easy identification of needed items. The best technique and one that is used by the military, EMS agencies, operating suites, and emergency departments across the United States is to keep like items together (e.g. wound management supplies in one section/sub-container). Storing items in separate plastic sealable bags allows quick identification of items and helps to protect dry items from liquids. A more in-depth discussion regarding organization of kit contents can be found in Chapter 4: Building Your Kit.

Examples of First Aid Kit Containers

The most common types of containers fall into the following three categories and the next section will focus on the pros and cons of each with respect to durability, protection from the elements, portability, and cost.

Hard-shell Containers – These containers are the most durable and can protect all contents, including ampules or other glass medication containers. High quality hard-shells can be water resistant or waterproof and provide good environmental protection from dust and dirt. These containers are often bulky and are not as portable as the other types. Additionally, good quality hard-shells can be expensive. Best Use: home-based first aid kits, RVs, or boats.

Soft-sided Cordura® or Nylon Containers – Soft cases, when made with Cordura® or a heavy-duty nylon can be very durable for most first aid contents except glass vials or ampules. They usually contain vinyl or plastic compartments within, and when combined with small sealable plastic bags, create a double barrier against moisture or dirt. These containers are usually very portable and are used for most outdoor first aid kits. The US military and EMS agencies across the country use larger soft-side cases when working in the field. These cases can range in cost depending upon the organization, pockets, and inner material. Best use: automobile, travel, off-road vehicles, snowmobiles.

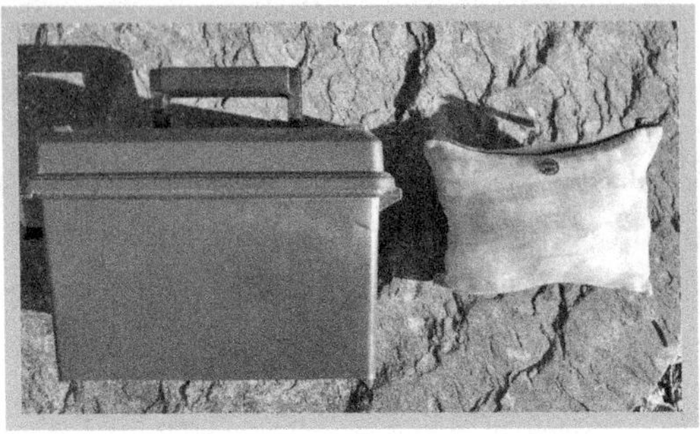

Examples of hard and soft-sided containers adapted for first aid kits.

Plastic Sealable Bags – Even the highest quality sealable bags lag far behind the other container types for durability, though they can be reinforced. Many outdoor professionals use sealable bags for their kits and they counteract the relative lack of sturdiness by strengthening them using duct tape either at the seams or to cover the entire bag. As long as the integrity of the bag remains true, it can protect items from moisture and dirt, especially if combined with additional smaller sealable bags within. Kits housed in these bags are as portable as other more durable soft-sided containers, but again, more care should be taken due to the thinness of material. Even with the purchase of a reflective, red, or orange duct tape to cover the outer parts of the bag, this is still the cheapest of the three options. Best use: automobile, personal travel, outdoor travel, off-road vehicles, snowmobiles.

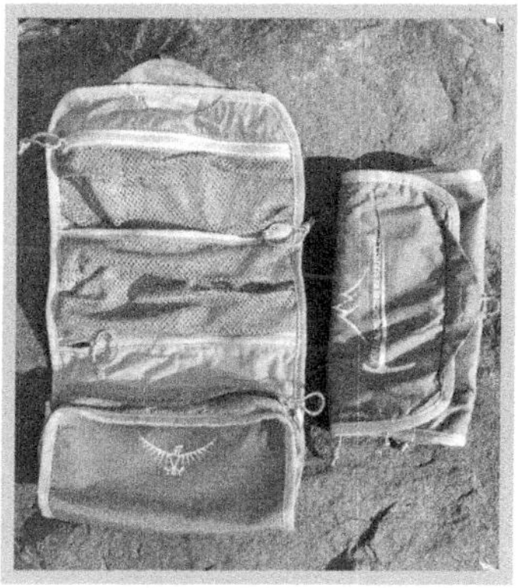

This kit bag, developed by Vertical Medicine Resources for use in the wilderness, has a number of compartments that can help to organize a first aid kit.

References

1. U.S. Department of Labor. Occupational Safety and Health Administration. American National Standards Institute/International Safety Equipment Association. *ANSI/ISEA Z308.1-2015. American National Standard Minimum Requirements for Workplace First Aid Kits and Supplies*. 2015.

4

Building Your Kit

Building Your Kit

It is impossible to be prepared for every conceivable emergency, but it is possible to be solution oriented and ready for the most common threats to your health and welfare. The purpose of this chapter is to provide a framework to select items to stock first aid kits for home and auto. Having identified the most common risks of injury in Chapter 2 and learned about best location, design, and organization of these kits, we are now ready to discuss common items that should be included.

While there are many methods that can be used when determining how to stock a kit, one of the most comprehensive to date was developed by the University of Utah School of Medicine in conjunction with a wilderness medicine organization called AdventureMed. Their mnemonic, PAWS, is simple and allows a systematic approach for the selection and organization of first aid kit components.

The mnemonic "PAWS" stands for:

P Prevention/Procedures
A Analgesics/Antibiotics/Antiseptics*
W Wound Care
S Survival[1]

While there are no government guidelines of appropriate items for inclusion into first aid kits for the home or in a vehicle, there are a number of organizations and hospitals that offer some guidance. The following sample content lists have been created after a review of this guidance, recent medical literature pertaining to first aid kit composition, and taking into account some of the guidelines for workplace first aid kits as listed in ANSI/ISEA regulation (ANSI/ISEA Z308 1-2015) referenced earlier. A reference list is included at the end of this chapter.[2-10]

P – Prevention and Procedures

Prevention

As Benjamin Franklin once said to his fellow Philadelphians in reference to fire safety in the city at the time, "An ounce of prevention is worth a pound of cure." The adage is equally true when considering the prevention of injury versus the treatment of injury. Preventative items make up a large percentage of most first aid kit contents and begin with basic items that might be easily overlooked.

All kits should include some type of alcohol-based hand sanitizer and/or soap, as well as at least two pairs of hospital exam gloves (these do not have to be sterile) for the prevention of disease spread and as a protective barrier against blood and other body fluids. Additionally, some type of breathing barrier (with a one-way valve) should be included within kits to allow for safe administration of breaths during cardiopulmonary resuscitation (CPR). Preventative items recommended by numerous organizations include:

Alcohol based hand sanitizer (or soap)
Breathing protective barrier (for CPR)
Disposable exam gloves (minimum of 2 pair)
Insect repellent
Heat pack/hand warmer (disposable)
Lip balm
Sunscreen
Sunglasses

Procedures

While the term sounds as if it would require a surgeon, "procedures" is primarily focused on completing very basic care such as removing a splinter or tick with a tweezer, taking a temperature, or perhaps measuring blood pressure. This category also includes equipment and instruments to fashion bandages, splint sprains, and clean wounds. Procedural items recommended by numerous organizations include:

Cold packs – for care of sprains/strains
Knife – small, always useful (also multi-tool)

Nail Clippers – trimming nails, dead skin
Safety pins – for use with triangular bandage/removal of splinters
Splint, aluminum – to temporarily splint sprains and fractures
Scissors/Shears – to cut tape, remove clothing, fashion bandages
Syringe/Turkey baster – to clean/flush wounds (see wound care)
Thermometer – to assess body temperature
Tweezers – for removal of splinters/small foreign bodies/ticks

A – Analgesics/Antibiotics/Antiseptics

Medications within a first aid kit will primarily consist of easy to acquire over the counter (OTC) medications. Prescription medications will likely be used on a regular basis and are generally stored in an easily accessible location within a bathroom or if temperature control is needed, in a refrigerator. Only during travel will these medications be commonly co-located within a first aid kit. The three categories listed below are the most common types of OTC medications included within first aid kits.

(*The fourth category on the list is *anaphylaxis*. Though not an OTC medication, epinephrine is included here for families with members who have severe allergies and are prescribed this medication via auto-injector.)

• • •

Analgesics

Analgesics is a group of drugs used to achieve pain relief (analgesia).

Acetaminophen
Aspirin (81 mg; do not give to children, for use during suspected heart attack or for other pain)
Ibuprofen (or Naproxen)

Antibiotics

Antibiotics is a group of drugs used to kill or slow the growth of bacteria. These drugs treat bacterial infections, not viruses.

Antibiotic ointment (bacitracin or triple antibiotic)
Other antibiotics (by prescription only)

Antiseptics

Antiseptics are substances that reduce or stop the growth of potentially harmful microorganisms on the skin.

Alcohol wipes
Antiseptic towelettes
Hydrogen peroxide
Providone iodine

***Anaphylaxis**

Epinephrine via auto-injector (these should be carried at

all times for individuals with known severe allergies) or needle-and-syringe.

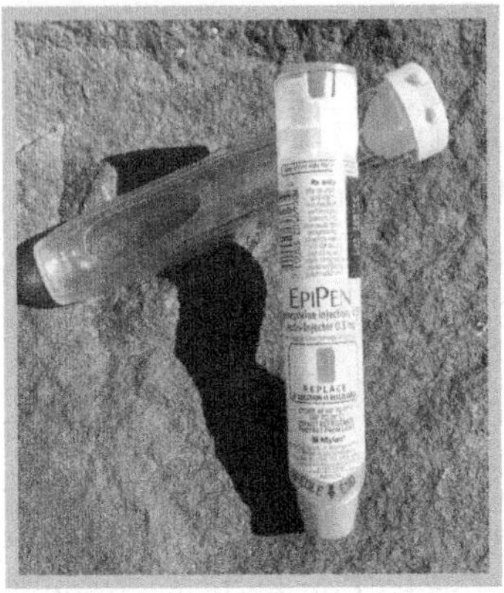

One type of epinephrine auto-injector.

Other medications to consider

Aloe Vera gel – for sunburns
Antacid (aluminum hydroxide and simethicone, etc.)
Anti-diarrhea medication (loperamide, bismuth subsalicylate)
Antihistamine – for allergies, bee/insect sting (diphenhydramine)
Calamine – for poison ivy/oak
Cold/cough medication (guaifenesin etc.)
Eye drops/eye wash solution
Hydrocortisone cream (1%)
Laxative
Oral re-hydration salts (ORS)

Petroleum jelly/other lubricant
Sting relief pad (topical lidocaine)

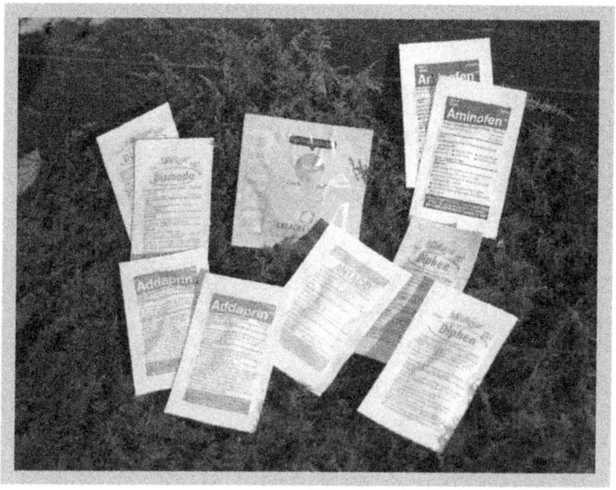

Single dose packaging of medications saves space.

W – Wound Care

Caring for injuries often requires substantial amounts of bandages and a wide variety of sizes and shapes is highly recommended. Abrasions are the most common types of wound and one of the most common injuries suffered. Luckily, they require little more than a good cleaning to remove debris and covering using a non-adherent dressing (one that does not "stick" to the wound). Lacerations are also common in the household, especially the kitchen and many minor lacerations can be adequately cared for at home with a well-supplied kit. As with all accidents at home—the first aid kit is meant to bridge the gap between onset of illness or injury and the arrival of trained EMS professionals or a visit to the emergency department. The components listed below will address almost every type of wound sustained in a home environment:

Adhesive bandages (assorted sizes)
Adhesive tape (cloth or silk)
Cotton-tipped applicators
Elastic wrap bandages (3 in. "ace" wrap)
Moleskin
Non-adherent sterile gauze pads (3x3 or 4x4)
Skin glue
Sterile gauze pads (3x3 and 4x4)
Syringe (to flush wounds)
Tourniquet (if trained—for severe arterial bleeding to limb)
Transparent dressing
Triangular bandages (for sling or compression)
Wound closure strips

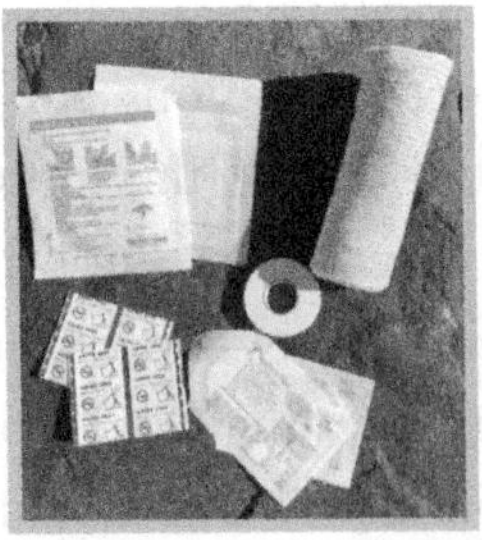

A first aid kit should contain various types of wound care items.

S – Survival

Though it may sound incongruous to include survival as a category for a first aid kit, there are many items that will help when our modern conveniences of electricity, heat, and communication are disrupted. An ice storm can drop trees onto power lines, a flood can close roads, and greater natural disasters such as tornados, hurricanes, and earthquakes can disrupt or destroy the infrastructure needed to care for our families adequately. Consider the region where you live and take into account weather phenomena that might affect your ability to care for your family. The items below may help "weather" whatever may come your way:

Butane lighter
Candles
Dust mask
Extra batteries
Extra blankets
Extra food/water
Flashlight or headlamp
Multi-tool
Solar Charger for cell phone and electronics
Space blanket
Toilet paper
Waterproof matches
Water purification tablets
Whistle

Emergency Information

There are a few additional important items to keep with your first aid kit at home and in your vehicle. They include a flashlight, a first aid manual, medical information for your family, and a list of emergency phone numbers.

Having a flashlight or headlamp, along with extra batteries is a good idea to keep co-located with your family's first aid kits. Make sure to check battery life each time you check your first aid kit for expired items. A good time to do this is with the time change twice a year.

No matter how much you were taught in your first aid class, in an emergency situation it is easy to forget a step or not remember a key item. Keep the first aid manual with your kit and it will be readily available when that emergency occurs.

One of the best things you can do in an emergency is to have basic medical information for all of your family members included with your first aid kit. Having this information readily available for EMS when they arrive (see an example list below) will speed their ability to quickly and competently care for your loved one and pass along important medical information to health care providers in the local emergency department.

Name:
Sex:
Birthdate:

Height (inches):
Weight (pounds):
Allergies (and reaction):
Previous Medical History:
Previous Surgical History:
Any information and timing of current illness/injury:

The final items to co-locate with your first aid kit are contact information and emergency phone numbers. All of this can be found on a phone, but would it not be better to have it readily available? Contact information should include family physician, pediatrician, any specialty care providers, local emergency services, and the poison control line. In the United States, the American Association of Poison Control Centers (AAPCC) phone number is available 24 hours/365 days a year at **(800) 222-1222.**

Disease and Condition Specific Considerations

If someone in your family suffers from a known condition such as heart disease, diabetes, or anaphylaxis, it is important to augment your kit with additional items to provide for that condition. Even something as simple as a contact lens container, additional contact lens solution, or a spare set of glasses can make a world of difference in an emergency or disaster situation. Items to consider based upon family needs are:

Blood glucose monitor
Diabetes testing supplies

Epinephrine auto-injector
Glucose tablets

How to Purchase Items for your First Aid Kit

As discussed in the introduction, first aid kits can often be assembled for a fraction of the cost of a commercially available kit. To find the best prices for kit containers, it is best to shop at retail department or home improvement stores or look at online first aid supply retailers or Amazon.com/Alibaba.com. While you can acquire items very inexpensively at Alibaba.com you must be very careful of quality at this retailer.

For kit contents, avoid drugstores as the prices at these locations are generally much more expensive than at big box retail stores, discount department stores, and online options. Many online first aid supply and surplus goods retailers have frequent sales. With a little patience and a well-considered supply list, stocking a kit can be kept inexpensive.

Finally, pay close attention to expiration dates of items, especially medications. Try to find items with the furthest expirations possible. In some cases, it may make sense to pay more for an item with a longer period before expiration.

Discount Retailers

I have found quality items in the following retailers when building first aid kits or finding containers for these kits.

Harbor Freight Tools – a great store for waterproof and other hard-sided containers

Big Lots – as with many of these retailers, stock is constantly changing, so check often

Ollie's Bargain Outlet – great finds in bandages and OTC medications

Any of the "dollar" stores – careful hunting can identify good bargains

Online Retailers

Some examples of online retailers that specifically market and sell first aid items are included below. The key with these websites is to look at the "per unit cost" as many of these retailers sell in bulk quantities.

First Aid Store
first-aid-store.com
Mfasco Health and Safety
www.mfasco.com
Emergency Medical Products
www.buyemp.com/category/first-aid

References

1. Della-Guistina D, Ingebretsen, R. *Advanced Wilderness Life Support*. 9th ed. Utah: AdventureMed, 2016.

2. American Red Cross. Make a First Aid Kit. Available

at: www.redcross.org/get-help/how-to-prepare-for-emergencies/anatomy-of-a-first-aid-kit.html. Accessed January 30, 2019.

3. Quinn R, Wedmore I, Johnson E, Islas A, Anglim A, Zafren K, Bitter C, Mazzorana V. Wilderness Medical Society practice guidelines for basic wound management in the austere environment: 2014 update. *Wilderness Environ Med.* 2014; 118-133.

4. Leeman D, Schimelpfenig T. Wilderness injury, illness, and evacuation: National Outdoor Leadership School's Incident Profiles, 1999-2002. *Wilderness Environ Med.* 2003; 14:174-182.

5. Griffiths R, Fernandez R, Ussia C. Is tap water a safe alternative to normal saline for wound irrigation in the community setting? *J Wound Care.* 2001; 10:407-411.

6. Gentile D, Morris J, Schimelpfenig T, Bass S, Auerbach P. Wilderness injuries and illnesses. *Annals of Emerg Med.* 1992; 21(7): 853-61.

7. U.S. Department of Labor. Occupational Safety and Health Administration. American National Standards Institute/International Safety Equipment Association. *ANSI/ISEA Z308.1-2015. American National Standard Minimum Requirements for Workplace First Aid Kits and Supplies.* 2015.

8. U.S. Department of Labor. Occupational Safety and Health Administration. Occupational Safety and Health Standards. First-aid Kits (Mandatory). Electronic Code

of Federal Regulations 1910.266 App A. Available at: www.osha.gov/laws-regs/regulations/standardnumber/1910/1910.266AppA. Accessed January 30, 2019.

9. Johnson TD. Tips for creating a useful first aid kit. *The Nation's Health*. April 2012; 42(3):24.

10. American Red Cross. Survival Kit Supplies. Available at: www.redcross.org/get-help/how-to-prepare-for-emergencies/survival-kit-supplies.html. Accessed January 31, 2019.

5

Sample Kit Contents

(PERSONAL, HOME, AUTO)

Sample Kit Contents (Personal, Home, Auto)

As mentioned in Chapter 4, there are no government recommendations for appropriate items for first aid kits for home and auto, though multiple non-profit organizations, hospitals, and medical researchers have created lists of appropriate items to be considered. Based on all of this information, the content lists below include all consensus items from these sources. All of the kit contents are organized using the PAWS acronym described in Chapter 4. Again, recommendations listed here are meant to be used as examples from which to develop your own customized kits that are best suited for you, your family, your environment, and your personal circumstance.

Personal First Aid

This is a small one-person kit, stored ideally in a soft-sided nylon bag, that can be used when traveling for business or pleasure. This kit will usually contain primarily preventative items, common medications (both OTC and prescription), and basic wound care supplies. If used while traveling overseas, be sure to consult the US Centers for Disease Control Traveler's Health website at wwwnc.cdc.gov/travel/destinations/list/ to identify any vaccinations or medications needed due to endemic disease in a country or region. The recommended packing list below includes an amount of each item in parentheses. Adjust these numbers to your personal comfort level. Please consult manufacturer packaging for proper dosing of all medications.

P – Prevention/Procedure

(2) Disposable exam gloves
(1) Sunscreen – small tube or multiple foil packets
(1) Sunglasses
(1) Lip balm – with SPF factor
(1) Insect repellant – small spray bottle
(?) Malaria prophylaxis (if traveling to endemic regions)

A – Analgesics/Antibiotics/Antiseptics

All quantities below provide 24-hour coverage for one adult.

(8) Acetaminophen (325 mg) – relief of pain and fever

(4) Antacid (type dependent) – relief of stomach upset, indigestion, heartburn
(1) Bacitracin/triple antibiotic ointment – one tube or multiple foil
(8) Diphenhydramine (25 mg) – temporary relief of allergies
(1) Epinephrine auto-injector – if prescribed
(12) Ibuprofen (200 mg) – relief of aches, pains
(8) Loperamide (2 mg) – anti-diarrheal
(?) Personal vitamins – as desired
(?) Prescription medications – as needed

W – Wound Care

(12) Adhesive bandages (assorted sizes)
(4) Sterile gauze pads (3x3)
(4) Sterile alcohol pads
(1) Adhesive tape – 0.5 in. silk or cloth

S – Survival

(?) Extra food, clothing, water as necessary
(1) Headlamp
(1) Small knife or multi-tool – remove from carry-on luggage!

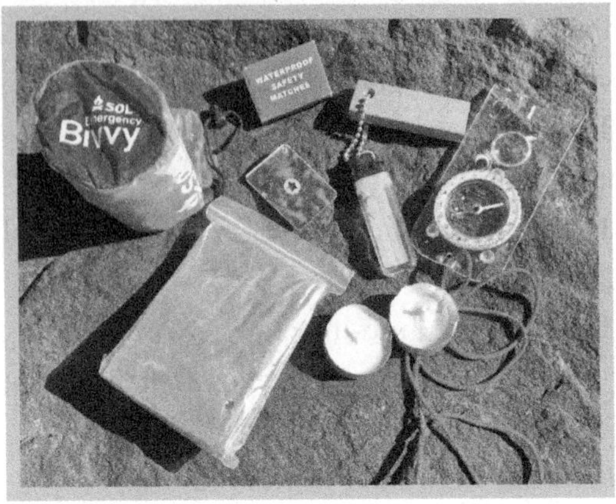

Common survival items include fire starting materials, signaling devices, and emergency blankets.

Home First Aid Kit

As described in Chapter 4, a home based first aid kit should be larger than a personal kit for travel. This kit should include a more comprehensive range of all medications and wound care supplies and a number of procedural items. The recommendations below are based on two adults. Adjust quantities after assessing household risks and number of persons who will be treated using the kit. The recommended packing list below includes an amount of each item in parentheses. Adjust these numbers to your personal comfort level. Please consult manufacturer packaging for proper dosing of all medications.

. . .

P – Prevention/Procedure

(1) Alcohol based hand sanitizer – one bottle or multiple foil packets
(1) Breathing protective barrier
(4) Disposable exam gloves
(1) Insect repellent – one bottle, place in plastic bag to prevent spillage
(4) Heat pack/hand warmer – two for each family member
(1) Lip balm – with SPF
(1) Sunscreen – one bottle or multiple foil packets
(1) Sunglasses – can be kept separate
(2) Cold packs
(1) Knife/multi-tool
(1) Nail clippers – large
(10) Safety pins – medium/large sizes
(1-2) Splint, aluminum – ideally two sizes (4 in. & 36 in.)
(1) Scissors – trauma shears if possible
(1) Syringe/Turkey baster
(1) Thermometer – oral
(1) Tweezers

A – Analgesics/Antibiotics/Antiseptics

All quantities below provide three days of coverage for one adult based upon standard manufacturers guidelines for dosages.

(24) Acetaminophen (325 mg) – relief of pain and fever
(1) Aloe Vera gel – topical treatment of abrasions, minor burns
(2) Antiseptics – wipes and liquid (See Appendix A for types)
(12) Antacid (type dependent) – relief of stomach upset, indigestion, heartburn
(12) Aspirin (81 mg) – relief of pain, fever; use with heart attack victims
(1) Bacitracin/triple antibiotic ointment – one tube or multiple foil
(1) Calamine – bottle, relief from poison ivy/oak, itching
(?) Cold/cough medication – personal choice
(24) Diphenhydramine (25 mg) – temporary relief of allergies
(1) Eye drops/eye wash solution – for eye irritation, removal of foreign body
(1) Epinephrine auto-injector – if prescribed
(1) Hydrocortisone cream (1%) – relief of skin irritation, one tube or multiple foil
(?) Laxative – (sennoside, doculate sodium) softening of stool
(36) Ibuprofen (200 mg) – relief of aches, pains (or Naproxen)
(24) Loperamide (2 mg) – anti-diarrheal
(2) Oral re-hydration salts (ORS) (electrolyte salts and glucose)
(1) Petroleum jelly/other lubricant – relief of skin irritation/diaper rash

(?) Personal vitamins – as desired

(?) Prescription medications – as needed

(1) Topical lidocaine – insect sting relief; one tube or multiple foils

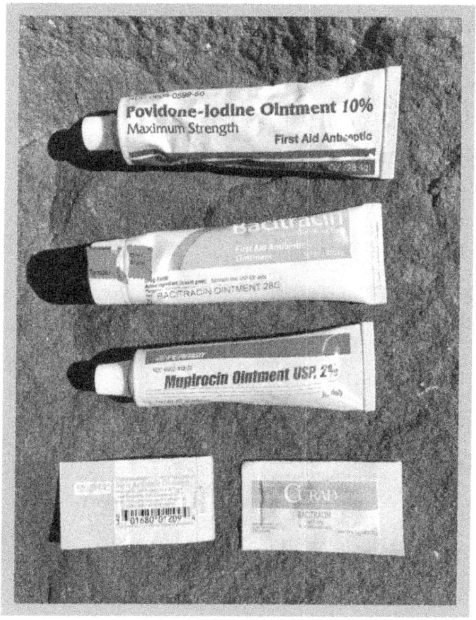

Various types of antibiotic creams for use on wounds. Note the smaller foil packs. These can save significant space and are useful for smaller kits.

W – Wound Care

(30) Adhesive bandages – medium/large sizes

(1) Adhesive tape – 0.5 in. cloth or silk

(20) Alcohol wipes

(2) Compression bandages – high absorption

(10) Cotton-tipped applicators
(1-2) Elastic wrap bandages – 3 in. recommended
(1) Moleskin – for blister/wound protection, cut to fit
(4) Non-adherent sterile gauze pads – assorted sizes
(1) Skin glue – one tube or multiple single use
(10) Sterile gauze pads – assorted sizes
(1) Syringe – for flushing wounds
(1) Tourniquet – if trained, for severe bleeding
(4) Transparent dressing – 3.5 in. x 4.125 in.
(1) Triangular bandages
(2) Wound closure strips – 0.5 in.

S – Survival

(1) Butane lighter – disposable
(4-8) Candles – consider one per room
(2) Dust mask – one per person
(4) Extra batteries – each size needed in household (AAA, AA, 9 volt)
(2) Extra blankets – wool blankets are warm and durable
(?) Extra food/water – personal preference
(2) Flashlight or headlamp – one per person
(1) Multi-tool
(1) Solar charger for electronics – with applicable cables
(2) Space blanket
(2) Toilet paper – rolls

(1) Waterproof matches – one box
(?) Water purification tablets – minimum five day supply
(1) Whistle

Auto First Aid Kit

First aid kits for automobiles should focus on providing minimal medications for common passengers, well-stocked wound care items in case of a motor vehicle crash, and survival items in case of accidental stranding due to weather or maintenance. The recommended packing list below include an amount of each item in parentheses. Adjust these numbers to your personal comfort level. Please consult manufacturer packaging for proper dosing of all medications.

P – Prevention/Procedure

(1) Alcohol based hand sanitizer – one bottle or multiple foil packets
(1) Breathing protective barrier – collapsible, high quality
(2) Disposable exam gloves
(2) Heat pack/hand warmer
(1) Lip balm – with SPF
(1) Sunscreen – one bottle or multiple foil packets
(1) Sunglasses – per passenger
(1) Cold packs
(1) Knife/multi-tool/glass break/seatbelt cutter
(1) Splint, aluminum – 36 in.
(1) Scissors – trauma shears if possible

A – Analgesics/Antibiotics/Antiseptics

All quantities below provide a single dose of coverage for one adult based upon standard manufacturers guidelines for dosages.

(2) Acetaminophen (325 mg) – relief of pain and fever
(2) Antiseptics – wipes and liquid (See Appendix A for types)
(4) Aspirin (81 mg) – relief of pain, fever; use with heart attack victims
(1) Bacitracin/triple antibiotic ointment – one tube or multiple foil
(2) Diphenhydramine (25 mg) – temporary relief of allergies
(1) Eye drops/eye wash solution – for eye irritation, removal of foreign body
(1) Epinephrine auto-injector – if prescribed
(4) Ibuprofen (200 mg) – relief of aches, pains (or Naproxen)
(2) Loperamide (2 mg) – anti-diarrheal
(?) Prescription medications – as needed

W – Wound Care

(30) Adhesive bandages – medium/large sizes
(1) Adhesive tape – 0.5 in. cloth or silk
(20) Alcohol wipes
(4) Compression bandages – high absorption

(1-2) Elastic wrap bandages – 3 in. recommended
(4) Non-adherent sterile gauze pads – assorted sizes
(1) Skin glue – one tube or multiple single use
(10) Sterile gauze pads – assorted sizes
(1) Syringe – for flushing wounds
(1) Tourniquet – if trained, for severe bleeding
(4) Transparent dressing – 3.5 in. x 4.125 in.
(1) Triangular bandages
(2) Wound closure strips – 0.5 in.

S – Survival

(1) Butane lighter – disposable
(2) Candles
(2) Dust mask
(4) Extra batteries – for flashlight/headlamp
(1) Extra blanket – wool blankets are warm and durable
(?) Extra food/water – personal preference
(1) Flashlight or headlamp – one per person
(1) Multi-tool (see within prevention/procedure)
(1) Solar charger for electronics – with applicable cables
(2) Space blanket
(1) Toilet paper – rolls
(1) Waterproof matches – one box
(2) Water purification tablets (depending on kind)
(1) Whistle

6

Safety Contents for Vehicles

Safety Contents for Vehicles

In addition to a comprehensive and personalized first aid kit, there are a number of safety items that are useful to keep in the vehicle at all times. This includes gear in case of an automotive breakdown or natural disaster and subsequent stranding. Having additional warm clothing, gloves, and a beanie for the winter is a smart precaution, especially when driving long distances in areas known for winter weather patterns that can produce large amounts of precipitation quickly. Extra food and water (and toilet paper!) are nice to have on any occasion, but making a habit of having some water, a few pre-packaged snack items, and some toilet paper can make an enormous difference in comfort if stranded overnight. Of course, limit water or liquid storage in a vehicle when the temperatures flirts with freezing.

Another item that is highly recommended is a combination seat belt cutter/window break device. This item will allow easier escape in the event of an automobile fire, entrapment after an accident, or accidental submerging (as electric windows don't operate well when exposed to water). This item should be stored in the glovebox or storage compartment in the passenger cabin and within reach of the driver and passengers.

In areas with cold climates, a wool blanket, space blankets, or even a large plastic garbage bag will help trap heat. A candle (or two) with matches or a lighter can raise the temperature in a closed vehicle by many degrees.

The list below includes some items that are useful to store in a vehicle depending on location and season (along with possible uses). Some of these items should be no surprise and are commonly included in all new vehicles sold.

Item (with possible uses)

Bungee cords – to keep a trunk closed or piece of fender after an accident
Cell phone charger – lighter or solar
Charger cables – to jump-start a battery
Collapsible shovel – in case of a stuck tire in snow
Extra bottle of engine oil – low oil
Fire extinguisher – for engine fires
Ice scraper – to remove ice, snow
Map or atlas – for directional aid
Plastic tarp – for laying on during repairs

Road flares/triangle – for signaling
Sand or cat litter – for better tire traction, weight over rear wheels
Spare tire and jack – to replace a flat tire
Tire chains – if in a snowy region
Tool kit – for minor fixes
Zip ties – used to temporarily hold items in place

Considerations for other forms of transportation

While family cars, SUVs, and trucks are most common on the interstates and highways of the United States, there are a number of other specialty forms of transportation that require different considerations including recreational vehicles, boats, aircraft, off-road vehicles, and snowmobiles. Each of these are discussed below.

Recreational Vehicles and Travel Trailers

Recreational vehicles (RV) continue to be popular with over 500,000 travel trailers, motorhomes, and folding camping trailers sold in 2017 and an estimated total of 9 million currently on the road.[1-2] There is even a social media fed subculture called "van-life" that is attracting young people who work from the road and are "location independent." This type of vehicle requires a first aid kit that combines the aspects of a home kit and a vehicle kit. RVs range in size from tractor-trailer and bus sized units to smaller vans and folding camping trailers. The size of the first aid kit can be limited based upon the size of the unit, but keeping a dedicated kit for this vehicle is a smart move. There are no specific risks related to RV use beyond that of a normal vehicle, but "home" aspects like cooking and associated injuries (lacerations) should be considered when developing a kit for an RV. An environmental risk to consider include potential for burns from campfires or incorporated cooking stoves.

Boats

Boating continues to be a popular pastime in the United States and Canada and depending on the kind of boating you do (sailing, canoeing, rafting, or kayaking) there is additional potential for injury. No matter the type of watercraft, these kits must be contained and compartmentalized in waterproof containers.

As with RVs mentioned above, the size of the kit is dependent, not only on activity, but also on the size of the vessel. A canoe or kayak first aid kit will be much different in size, scope, and contents than a first aid kit for a cabin cruiser or small yacht. Keep in mind the common dangers for each and the size limitations when developing kits.

Drowning is the most obvious concern in aquatic environments. Preventative measures, such as knowing how to swim and ensuring that all persons on a boat are wearing a life jacket, are essential.[3-4] Drowning was the third leading cause of unintentional injury death in 2017. Seasickness is another concern and dimenhydrinate is an obvious OTC medication to add to boat first aid kits. Playing in and around water can lead to chapped hands and so a lanolin-based hand cream would be useful as would a larger supply of sunscreen.

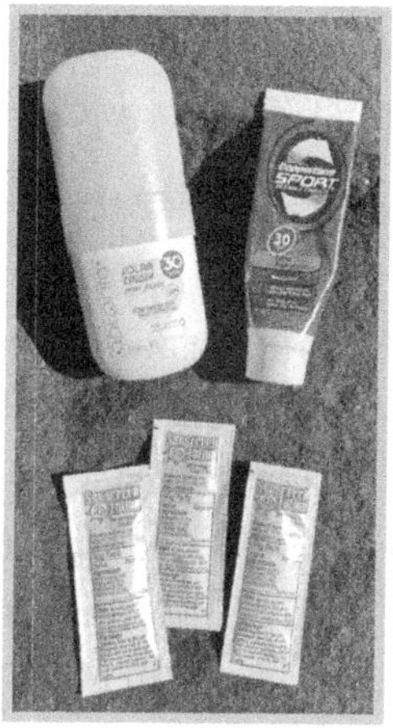

Sunscreen is an essential item for waterborne first aid kits.

Recreational scuba diving, independently or on a commercial dive boat, adds another level of risk to consider. Diving injuries require specialized knowledge and equipment and include such things as decompression illness, drowning, barotrauma, head injury, shark attack, rope/propeller injuries, and aquatic animal bites and stings. Before booking with any commercial dive company, it is important to ask these three questions:

Does the dive boat hold a well-stocked first-aid kit that is regularly checked and replenished?

Does the dive boat hold adequate emergency oxygen and appropriate oxygen delivery equipment?

Does the dive boat have a crew member trained in dive rescue, first-aid and oxygen provision?[5]

Aircraft

According to the Federal Aviation Administration (FAA) there are approximately 166,000 fixed wing recreational aircraft and over 10,000 rotary wing aircraft (helicopters) plying the skies of the United States each year. While aircraft accidents are rare in the commercial industry, accidents do occur each year with recreational aircraft. The FAA has devised regulations on first aid training and kits for commercial carriers but no such guidelines exist for private aircraft.[6] Additionally, the International Civil Aviation Organization (ICAO) has developed a minimum standard of first aid kit contents for commercial carriers. A study, conducted in 2010, compared the first aid kits of 12 airlines and found that none of them met these guidelines.[7] The study recommended "that all national authorities increase their periodic checks to ensure that all airlines maintain complete and up-to-date emergency medical kits aboard their aircraft in order to increase passenger safety."[7] One additional note: although throughout this book we discuss the need for proper training to accompany first aid kits, this is not the case for commercial aircraft. Depending on the carrier, each aircraft carries a more advanced medical kit with equipment and medications that go beyond a standard layperson's ability. This is due to the likely potential of a medical doctor or other health professional being a passenger and their ability to render care while airborne utilizing the included advanced gear and medications.

Having a first aid kit and associated emergency supplies is a must have for owners of fixed and rotary wing aircraft, especially considering the potential remoteness of an accident site. These kits should be fairly robust in contents, particularly in the wound care and survival components as an aircraft accident will likely result in traumatic injury with an unknown delay in rescue due to difficulties accessing the accident site. Pilots must evaluate these needs while also considering the size and especially, the weight of the kit contents for the particular airframe.

Off-Road Vehicles

Off-road vehicles include a number of motorized conveyances such as all-terrain vehicles (ATVs), utility task vehicles (UTVs), and off-road motorcycles. All of these have the ability to transport their riders far away from definitive medical care. As with other specialty vehicles, this class has specific injury patterns. There are approximately 500 deaths due to ATV accidents each year along with roughly 90,000 visits to emergency departments within the US due to ATV related injury.[8] Serious injuries are generally due to impact accidents and include traumatic head injuries, fractures, lacerations, and sprains that are typical to this type of incident. A first aid kit located in a bag or pannier is a prudent measure and should be carried. Kits should include a device to communicate to rescuers (cell phone, handheld radio, etc.), an accurate device to measure location (GPS), and wound care materials to splint fractures, care for sprains, and stop/control bleeding.

Snowmobiles

Snowmobiles are similar to off-road vehicles in terms of associated risk and injury patterns. Impact with terrain or man-made objects are the cause for most injuries though hypothermia and asphyxia due to burial from avalanches are two other concerns.[9] Snowmobilers account for the largest percentage of deaths from avalanche in the United States (23%) as measured between 1951-2013.[10] First aid kits should be well-equipped in wound care supplies in order to deal with traumatic injuries. Kits should also include extra warm/dry clothing and warming devices to counter hypothermia and communication devices (including avalanche beacons – ideally located on the rider) when venturing into avalanche prone terrain.

References

1. RV Industry Association (RVIA). Business Indicators 2017. Available at: www.rvia.org/business-indicators. Accessed January 31, 2019.

2. Marcus J. The RV industry has rebounded in a big

and beautiful way. *The Boston Globe*. Available at: www.-bostonglobe.com/lifestyle/travel/2016/06/02/the-industry-has-rebounded-big-and-beautiful-way/5CYTj7Ei5UbHbU3r2Zl80L/story.html. Accessed January 31, 2019.

3. Schmidt A, Sempsrott J, Hawkins SC. Special Report: The Myth of Dry Drowning Remains at Large. *Emergency Medicine News*. 2018; 40(6).

4. Schmidt A, Sempsrott JR, Hawkins SC, Cushing TA, Arastu A, Auerbach PS. Wilderness Medical Society Practice Guidelines for the Prevention and Treatment of Drowning. *Wilderness Environ Med.* 2016 Jun;27(2):236-251.

5. Pye J, Greenhalgh T. First aid kits for recreational dive boats, what should they contain? *Travel Med Infect Dis*. 2010; 8: 311-317.

6. Federal Aviation Administration. Regulations and Policies: AC 120-44A - Air Carrier First Aid Programs. Available at: www.faa.gov/regulations_policies/advisory_circulars/index.cfm/go/document.information/documentID/22766. Accessed February 6, 2019.

7. Sand M, Gambichler T, Sand D, et al. Emergency medical kits on board commercial aircraft: A comparative study. *Travel Med Infect Dis*. 2010; 8: 388-394.

8. Rattan R, Joseph AK, Dente CJ, et al. Prevention of all-terrain vehicle injuries: A systematic review from The

Eastern Association for the Surgery of Trauma. *Trauma Acute Care Surg*. 2018;84(6):1017-26.

9. Jekich BM, Drake BD, Nacht JY, et al. Avalanche Fatalities in the United States: A Change in Demographics. *Wilderness Environ Med*. 2016;27(1):46-52.

10. Van Tilburg C, Grissom CK, Zafren K, et al. Wilderness Medical Society Practice Guidelines for Prevention and Management of Avalanche and Nonavalanche Snow Burial Accidents. *Wilderness Environ Med*. 2017;28(1):23-42.

7

Storage, Care, and Inspection of Kits

Storage, Care, and Inspection of Kits

Assembling a first aid kit is just one of three important aspects of first aid preparedness along with long term maintenance of the kit and acquisition of first aid knowledge and practical skills. Storage, care, and inspection of kits periodically is a requirement to ensure that you have what is necessary when an emergency occurs.

Storage and Care

Many items in a first aid kit, especially medications, are sensitive to changes in temperature, humidity, and light. This can not only effect medications, but also the integrity of packaging for a variety of items within a first aid kit. The ideal environment to store a kit is one that is cool, dark, and dry. It must be accessible to adults and kept in a location where young children cannot accidentally gain access. Most medications should be stored at "room temperature," which is defined as 59-86° F (15-

30° C). Follow the manufacturer guidelines as listed on the packaging of each product.

Storage recommendations for select OTC medications

Acetaminophen – room temperature, avoid freezing, not light sensitive
Aloe Vera gel – avoid excessive heat and prolonged direct sunlight
Antacids – most at room temperature, do not freeze, protect from heat, light, and moisture
Ibuprofen – store at room temperature and protect from light
Laxatives – avoid excessive heat and prolonged direct sunlight

Inspection

Always inspect first kits on a regular basis. Twice a year is optimal. A good technique to adopt is to conduct this check in the Fall and Spring when the time changes. This always occurs on a weekend and is the same recommendation as is promoted to change batteries in smoke detectors and check the function of fire extinguishers.

Focus on two areas when inspecting a first aid kit: 1) Expiration dates of medications and supplies and 2) the integrity of all packaging. If in doubt about the sterility or integrity of any item, replace it!

. . .

Other Care Tips

- Consider adding a packet of desiccant to the first aid kit to decrease humidity within the container.

- Many medications need protection from sunlight. Store medications together in a dark colored re-sealable bag within the first aid kit.

- If storing medications outside of their original containers, label name and dosage on the new container. Save product information and dosage recommendations within the new container. Small re-sealable bags save space and can be labeled easily with tape or marker.

- Certain plastic, rubber, and latex products will break down over time. Carefully inspect these items for small cracks or tears.

- Periodically swap out alcohol and other antiseptic wipes as these can dry out over time.

8

Recommended Training

Recommended Training

A first aid kit is only as useful as the person holding it. Learning basic concepts of first aid takes little time but may pay enormous dividends in the case of an emergency. There are a number of training opportunities available for the layperson in basic first aid and cardiopulmonary resuscitation (CPR). These courses are generally held on the evenings or weekends and are relatively inexpensive. All of the courses discussed below award certification in the training provided. Certification is usually for a two-year period and requires either retaking the full course or completing a refresher course to maintain certification. As with many fields of knowledge, medicine is constantly changing based on new evidence. Therefore, it is important to return for retraining regularly to stay current and to refresh skills learned previously.

The next level of training and preparedness is to enroll

in a wilderness first aid (WFA) or wilderness first responder (WFR) courses. Even if you are not an "outdoor person" these courses are useful in that they focus on providing care with limited resources, as would be the case in a disaster or weather-related incident.

The wilderness first aid course is geared to individuals who enjoy spending time in the outdoors, often at a great distance from medical assistance. A WFA course usually consists of 16 hours of instruction and is often offered over a weekend. The wilderness first responder course is geared to outdoor professionals such as camp counselors, guides, and outdoor trip leaders. The WFR is usually one week in length, goes into much more depth than any of the other courses and incorporates many hands-on learning activities.

Depending on the provider, these courses are offered in three forms: in person, blended learning, and online. As mentioned throughout the text, the importance of hands-on training using the tools and gear you have in your kit, is the most beneficial and has been proven as such in a number of studies. Many people don't have the time or the ability to attend in person classes. For these students, blended or online learning is more useful as some training is much better than no training!

In person – This type of course is delivered in a traditional classroom setting and allows maximal hands on training.

Blended – Blended training encompasses some work online, usually including videos and quizzes from the included literature. The online portion is self-paced and allows for less location dependence. In this format, you can work through the training as time allows and schedule a hands-on skill session after completing the online portion.

Online – All instruction is provided online and is usually self-paced, though some courses require attending virtual classes with other students. Online courses do not allow for any hands-on practice or work with a certified instructor.

American Red Cross (www.redcross.org)

The American Red Cross offers a variety of courses from basic CPR and first aid, to babysitting classes, and water safety/lifeguarding. The basic CPR, AED, and first aid courses are the most useful in delivering the knowledge necessary to effectively use a first aid kit in an emergency.

CPR – The cardiopulmonary resuscitation (CPR) course includes training in CPR for adults, children, and babies and is commonly combined with the AED class. ($75-$100 – combined with AED)

AED – AED is the commonly used initialism for automated external defibrillator. This course instructs the student in how to operate common commercial AEDs that are available in public places such as churches, malls, airports, and schools. It is usually combined with the CPR course. ($75-$100 – combined with CPR)

First Aid – This course is the most comprehensive offered by the American Red Cross as it often includes instruction in CPR and the use of an AED. It covers a wide range of emergencies that can occur at home or while traveling and includes asthma emergencies, anaphylaxis, burns, choking, diabetic issues, major bleeding and wound care, environmental emergencies, heart attacks, poisoning, injuries to the neck, head, and spine, stroke and seizure. ($100-125)

American Heart Association (www.heart.org)

While much of the training conducted by the American Heart Association is geared to medical professionals, the organization does provide courses to non-medically trained persons.

CPR/AED – The AHA's Heartsaver® CPR/AED class is available in the blended and in person settings. The cost for blended instruction is $15 for the online portion and approximately $75 for the hands-on training (varies by provider and group size). In person training costs between $75 and $100, again depending on provider and group size.

First Aid – The AHA also offers a first aid course and this program is usually combined with the CPR/AED instruction. It is available in blended and in person format and prices vary depending on provider and group size.

Wilderness Medicine Courses

The following wilderness medicine courses are an introduction to additional skills that are useful in emergencies, especially when away from home or when natural disasters strike. Wilderness medicine has been defined in the past based solely on distance from definitive care. Recently, two more accurate definitions are being used that better describe this type of care.[1-3]

Wilderness medicine is medical care delivered in those areas where fixed or transient geographic challenges reduce availability of, or alter requirements for, medical or patient movement resources.[1]

Wilderness medicine is medical care and problem-solving when the surrounding environment has, or has been allowed to have, more power over us than does the infrastructure (and underlying social structure) of our civilization.[1]

These definitions better describe the difficulties that can quickly mount when a layer of civilization such as electrical power, clean water delivery, on a disrupted road network are taken away. Wilderness medicine training takes first aid instruction to the next level by making students consider the difficulties of a limited resource environment where help may not be available for a significant amount of time for a variety of causes. These courses provide techniques to repurpose items into useful first aid equipment and more importantly, provides a framework for students to think outside the box in order to better care for their patients in less than ideal circumstances.

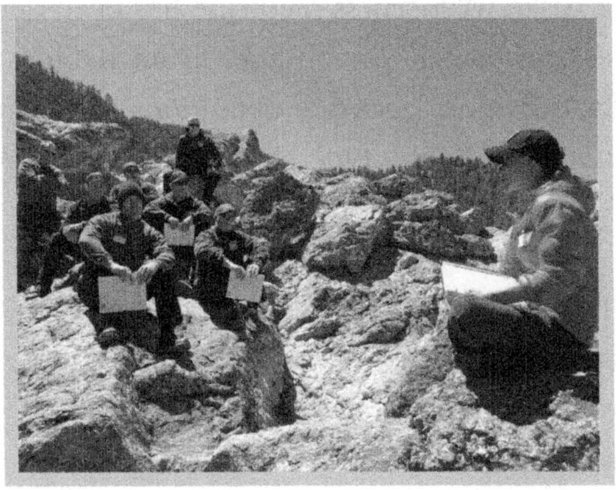

Wilderness medicine courses are often taught outside with hands-on practice scenarios.

Wilderness First Aid (WFA) – There is no set standard for instruction of WFA classes but generally these courses are delivered over 16 hours of instruction and are primarily classroom/outdoors based. It is the introductory course available in wilderness medicine and is highly recommended to build upon knowledge gained in standard first aid/CPR/AED training from the American Red Cross or the American Heart Association. The focus of these courses is primarily on prevention, recognizing signs and symptoms, and basic treatment options of common wilderness injuries and illnesses.

Advanced Wilderness First Aid (AWFA) or Wilderness Advanced First Aid (WAFA) is a similar course that is usually three days in length and discusses additional common injuries and treatment options. The areas below are commonly included in standard WFA courses:

WFA Topics

Patient assessment
Basic life support
Circulatory system issues
Acute Coronary Syndrome (ACS)
Respiratory system/airway
Nervous system issues
Spine injuries
Wounds
Burns
Musculoskeletal injuries
Allergic reactions
Anaphylaxis
Heat illness
Hypothermia
Lightning
Submersion
Common medical problems

Elective WFA Topics

Dislocations
Spine injury management
Local cold injury
Altitude Illness
Poisoning
Toxins: Snakebite
Toxins: Arthropods
Toxins: Marine[4]

Wilderness First Responder (WFR) – The wilderness first responder course is designed for the layperson and is normally six to eight days in length (70 hours of total training) and often include nighttime scenarios. It focuses on assessment and treatment of injuries or illness in a wilderness or remote setting where definitive care in not available. This course goes into greater depth than a WFA or an AWFA class and is often required of guides, summer camp counselors, and others in the outdoor industry. This training provides much more time for hands-on practical scenarios in wilderness environments. The following topics are commonly covered in some degree during a WFR course.

WFR Topics

Medical – Legal considerations
Blood borne pathogens
Patient assessment
Airway management

Shock
Wound management
Thermal burns
Sprains and strains
Fractures
Dislocations
Head and facial trauma
Spinal cord injuries
Chest trauma
Abdominal trauma
Lightning
Heat Injuries/dehydration
Cold Injuries
Hypothermia
Animal bites & stings
Poisons and toxins
Allergies and anaphylaxis
Altitude emergencies
Drowning
Water/food-borne Illness
Neuro emergencies
Respiratory distress
Chest pain
Abdominal pain
Genitourinary injury/illness
Diabetes
Expedition problems
Medical kits
Search and rescue
Packaging and transport
Stress management[5]

Wilderness Medicine Course Providers

There are dozens of companies that offer WFA and WFR courses across the United States. The list below includes some of the best from across the country along with their website address.

AdventureMed
www.awls.org
Aerie Backcountry Medicine
www.aeriemedicine.com
Hawk Ventures
www.hawkventures.com
Landmark Learning
www.landmarklearning.edu
NOLS Wilderness Medicine
www.nols.edu
Remote Medical International www.
remotemedical.com
Stonehearth Open Learning Opportunities
www.soloschools.com
Vertical Medicine Resources
www.vertical-medicine.com
Wilderness Medical Associates
www.wildmed.com

These companies, along with others, offer a host of different courses in addition to WFA and WFR. These include wilderness medicine courses aimed at medical professionals. Acronyms and initialisms abound for the names of these courses (WEMT, AWLS, WUMP, DiMM, etc.) and offer additional advanced skills and/or focus on a specific environment.

References

1. Hawkins SC. Introduction to Wilderness EMS. In Hawkins SC, ed. *Wilderness EMS*. Philadelphia, PA: Wolters Kluwer, 2018.

2. Sward DG, Bennett BL. Wilderness Medicine. *World J Emerg Med*. 2014;5(1):5-15.

3. McIntosh SE, Cushing TA, Keyes LE, Pollock NW. What is wilderness medicine? *Wilderness Environ Med*. 2015;26(1):1.

4. Johnson DE, Schimelpfenig T, Hubbell F. Minimum guidelines and scope of practice for wilderness first aid. *Wilderness Environ Med*. 2013;24(4):456-462.

5. Simon RB. Level of wilderness first aid training and knowledge retention of rock climbers in the United States. Master's Thesis, University of Leicester, 2016.

Epilogue

Having responded to emergencies in the United States and participated in rescues abroad, the one deciding factor that I have found along the razor's edge between life and death is preparation. Being prepared is not just a motto or a flippant quote on a Facebook post, but a way to move through life. Every day we prepare for small things... we brush our teeth, pack our lunches, make sure there is gasoline in the car, etc., but we often overlook preparation for big, though relatively uncommon things, such as accidents or unintentional injuries. It takes foresight and dedication to carve out time in a busy schedule to consider infrequent but potentially life changing possibilities. Doing so may make all the difference.

Too often after responding to an accident I have heard despondent family and friends of victims wish they had been able to do more to assist, to be able to make a difference, to help save their loved one. I am often asked what they could have done and my answer is always, "Be prepared with gear and training." Building a quality kit and getting basic first aid training are both very easy to accomplish but often difficult to start. By purchasing this book, you have taken the important first step to being ready for future emergencies and walking the razor's edge.

Appendix A: Common Over the Counter (OTC) Medication List (Generic and Brand Name)

Common Over the Counter (OTC) Medication List

Throughout the book, drugs are always referred to by their generic name in order to provide consistency, prevent confusion, and show no commercial bias to any manufacturer or product. The list within this appendix includes some of the most common OTC drugs that may be included within a first aid kit and their associated brand names. Inclusion within this appendix is not an endorsement of any product listed.

Common Over the Counter (OTC) Medications and Use

Generic name	Example Brand	Use
Acetaminophen	Tylenol	Pain, inflammation
Alcohol swabs		Topical antiseptic
Aloe Vera gel		Topical pain relief
Alumina magnesium	Maalox	Antacid
Aspirin	Disprin	Pain, inflammation
Bacitracin	Bacitracin	Topical antibacterial
Bacitracin-polymyxin b	Polysporin	Topical antibacterial
Bisacodyl	Dulcolax	Laxative
Bismuth subsalicylate	Pepto-Bismol	Antidiarrheal
Calamine		Topical anti-itch
Cetirizine	Zyrtec	Allergy/congestion
Cimetidine	Tagamet	Antacid
Diphenhydramine	Benadryl	Allergy/congestion
Dimenhydrinate	Dramamine	Motion sickness
Docusate sodium	Colace	laxative
Electrolyte solution	Pedialyte	Replace electrolytes
Epinephrine (Prescription)	EpiPen	Anaphylaxis
Eye drops	Artificial Tears	Eye care
Famotidine	Pepcid	Antacid
Fexofenadine	Allegra	Allergy/congestion
Guaifenesin	Mucinex	Cough and cold
Hydrocortisone cream (1%)	Cortisone 10	Topical anti-itch
Ibuprofen	Advil, Motrin	Pain, inflammation
Lidocaine		Topical pain relief
Lidocaine-benzalkonium chloride	Bactine	Topical pain relief
Loratadine	Claritin	Allergy/congestion
Loperamide	Imodium	Antidiarrheal
Naproxen	Aleve	Pain, inflammation
bacitracin-polymyxin b-neomycin	Neosporin	Topical antibacterial
Bacitracin-polymyxin b	Polysporin	Topical antibacterial*
Petroleum jelly	Vaseline	Skin irritation
Providone-iodine	Betadine	Topical antiseptic
Ranitidine	Zantac	Antacid
Sennosides	Senokot	Laxative

* Bacitracin-polymyxin b or bacitracin alone is likely preferable to bacitracin-polymyxin b-neosporin due to frequent allergies to neosporin.[1]

References

1. Hawkins SC, Simon RB, Beissinger JP, Simon D. *Vertical Aid: Essential Wilderness Medicine for Climbers, Trekkers, and Mountaineers*. New York: WW Norton, 2017.

Appendix B: Recommended Resources

Recommended Resources

There are a number of very good books on first aid and wilderness first aid available. Although no substitute for formal instruction, these guides are fantastic resources to refresh your knowledge or use in an emergency. Each listing includes the availability in e-book and print formats. Remember, keep your first aid guides with your kits for easy accessibility in an emergency.

Field Guide to Wilderness Medicine by PS Auerbach, B Constance, and L Freer – This thorough book, at 1008 pages, is still compact enough and highly recommended for inclusion in vehicles, but especially for aircraft, boats, or off-road vehicles that can transport you far away from medical help. (Print and e-book)

First Aid – This book, written in conjunction with the American Academy of Orthopaedic Surgeons (AAOS) and American College of Emergency Physicians (ACEP) covers basic first aid very well. (Print and e-book)

Vertical Aid: Essential Wilderness Medicine for Climbers, Trekkers, and Mountaineers by SC Hawkins, RB Simon, JP Beissinger, and D Simon – This book, though focusing on mountainous environments, is written for the layperson and includes all of the latest evidenced-based medicine available. (Print and e-book)

Wilderness & Travel Medicine – Written by E. Weiss, this book is a compact and useful manual to carry with a small personal kit or to keep in a vehicle. (Print and e-book)

There are also some very useful websites available that have links to training and what to do in an emergency.

American Heart Association – this link leads to the AHA CPR and First Aid training page.

www.heart.org/en/cpr

American Red Cross – this link leads to the organization's training and supplies page.

www.redcross.org/take-a-class

Mayo Clinic – this link leads to a first aid page that describes what to do in different types of medical emergencies.

www.mayoclinic.org/first-aid

Acknowledgments

It is with gratitude and appreciation that I acknowledge and thank my friends, colleagues, and mentors. Their passion, experience, and wisdom are unequaled in the field. I am grateful and want to extend my sincere thanks to: Seth C. Hawkins, MD; Pamela Holt, NP; J. Pearce Beissinger, PA-C; David Hillebrandt, MD; Linda Laskowski-Jones, MS, APRN; Corey Winstead, WEMT; and Tom Gall, EMT-P.

I especially want to thank my wonderful wife, Deb. Your love, support, and encouragement makes all the difference and brings more happiness than I deserve.

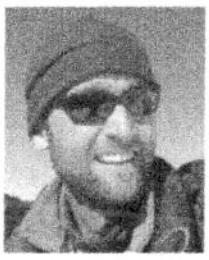

About the Author

R. Bryan Simon, RN, is a graduate of the United States Military Academy at West Point and a former US Army infantry officer and graduate of the US Army Ranger School. He is a Fellow in the Academy of Wilderness Medicine, a Master Fellow of the Adventurers and Explorers Guild, and holds a Diploma in Mountain Medicine from the UIAA. He is also a graduate of Radford University, has studied clinical nutrition at Cornell University, and has earned a master's degree in Mountain Medicine through the University of Leicester (UK).

Bryan serves on the editorial board for the journal *Nursing*, is the climbing medicine columnist for *Wilderness Medicine Magazine*, and is the senior editor for the American Alpine Club's yearly guide *Accidents in North American Climbing*. He writes on a variety of subjects related to nursing, first aid, and wilderness medicine. His work has been featured in magazines and journals such as *Emergency Medicine News*, *Critical Care Nursing*, and *Climbing*. He has also written *Hiking and Biking in the New River Gorge: A Trail User's Guide* (Wolverine Publishing) and is co-author of *Vertical Aid: Essential Wilderness Medicine for Climbers, Trekkers, and Mountaineers* (WW Norton).

Bryan has traveled around the world and has participated in rescues both here and abroad. He is a co-owner of the medical guiding company Vertical Medicine Resources (www.vertical-medicine.com), and serves on the board of directors for the Appalachian Mountain Rescue Team (AMRT) and the New River Alliance of Climbers (NRAC). Bryan is also the recipient of the 2014 Warren D. Bowman Award, presented for contributions in service to wilderness medicine and to the Wilderness Medical Society.

facebook.com/rbryansimon

twitter.com/RBryanSimon

Also by R. Bryan Simon

Vertical Aid: Essential Wilderness Medicine for Climbers, Trekkers, and Mountaineers (WW Norton)

Hiking and Biking in the New River Gorge: A Trail User's Guide (Wolverine Publishing)

Made in the USA
Monee, IL
04 November 2026

67384434R00059